The Lifestyle Overhaul Guide

Information based in reality,

Steeped in common sense and

Delivered painlessly

Table of Contents

Dedication: For Brandon. There are not enough pages to write an adequate dedication. Thank you for loving this crazy, free spirited, change monger.

Introduction

Change isn't easy. Most of the time, if people have to choose between keeping something the way it is or changing it they will choose to stay the same. I was told once that the status quo is the greatest enemy to innovators simply because the status quo always wins. It's when the status quo becomes unacceptable that people choose to change. This is especially true when we consider our health. "Don't fix what's not broken," is the turn of phrase most often used. The status quo wins. It is up to you to decide whether the status quo in your own life is acceptable. What has become unacceptable to you regarding your health? Consider the version of yourself when you felt at the top of your game. Have things changed? Is it acceptable to you to be reliant on prescriptions to stay well? Is it acceptable that not only is healthcare unaffordable, but the insurance that was meant to protect us from the unaffordable healthcare is now itself becoming unaffordable? Is this a status quo we can live with? I cannot. And, thus, I write.

While studying in chiropractic school, I was surrounded by others who had very similar belief systems. We understood the importance of a healthy nervous system, the necessity of doctors who care for you when we're sick and doctors who are there to keep us well. Above all, however, we simply could not understand how anyone else could think differently. Now that we're older and wiser, we call that, "Chiropractic Island." While in practice, you learn quickly that not everyone values your advice and might even think you're wrong: A tough pill to swallow for a new graduate at the time.

Over the years, I've come to realize that it isn't that my patients don't listen or are bad patients. Just as I had a limited sphere of understanding, so do they! You can only make decisions based on the information you've received. A huge part of my job as a doctor is simply sharing knowledge and I can honestly say, I learn more from my patients than I do from textbooks at times. I've been so fortunate to have an abundance of knowledge surrounding me with my father-in-law and husband both being chiropractors in different specialties. Having a family of chiropractors is cool to a degree I can't even begin to describe. My post-graduate work being done in pregnancy and pediatric, my husband's in sports rehabilitation and my father-in-law's in orthopedics. Talking shop at Thanksgiving, while annoying to everyone else, is something I've grown to love and appreciate. The region I practiced in Wisconsin was chock full of open-minded medical practitioners. They gave me insight into the world of allopathy I would have never known having had such a strong aversion to it in my earliest years of practice.

Chiropractors have a distinct and wonderful interpretation of how the body works and how to achieve optimal wellbeing. It is from within that we heal and where we begin each person's journey towards health.

Things are often thought of as happening *to* us when in fact they are happening *inside* us. Diving into research we find the same findings over and over that there really is no replacement to a healthy diet and regular exercise and that healing from within using those tools can have dramatic effects. The application and process by which people inject those things into their lives can vary greatly, be wildly expensive and be not nearly as effective as keeping it simple.

My mission is straight forward: To guide each individual on the easiest path towards health and give them the tools to help others do the same. There is one thing I know for sure and that is the United States is sick. We are sick from diseases that are 99% preventable. My job is to help you find your strength when met with indecision or weakness. I cannot promise you will lose a pound a day with this 90-day start-up, but I can promise you will have a new understanding and appreciation for the wonderment that is your body.

The truth is we *need* the United States to be healthier. With chronic diseases like Diabetes, cancer, heart disease, etc. on the rise, we spend more per capita on medical costs than any other country and are outperformed by many 3rd world countries in terms of our overall health. The economic burden of healthcare spending will bankrupt our country if nothing is done.

It is difficult, in the beginning, to feel connected to other people who are perfect strangers or to an issue that may not apply to you. After all, you have beliefs, routines, opinions, habits and relationships too. I ask only that you consider the choices of your actions, whether good or bad for your health, in the context of a community or greater entity. How will your smoking affect others?

Your family? How can your choices change the way a company produces goods? Can one person change their health and motivate others to change theirs and so on? Yes. We are in this together and we can help each other to great health. You don't have to go it alone.

Health is not simply the absence of disease or symptoms. Health is thriving, not just getting through another day. Health is kicking off the covers and hitting the ground running. Health is feeling your absolute best every single day and taking consistent action to be healthy. It is vibrancy and strength! It's a total package, not just lack of diagnoses.

What would happen if there was a widespread epidemic of health? Fewer people needing prescriptions? Less people going to urgent care? Less hospitalizations? How can your choices not only change the way we experience healthcare, but the health of other people? The answer is: in ways you cannot possibly predict! Turning the focus back on how to stay healthy versus how to treat conditions is a huge shift and unfamiliar paradigm to many, but a shift, if large enough, can alter large corporations and change policies. With a few changes, we can alter the course of healthcare.

What we all need is an easy and guided tour of the total health package. This is not a fad diet or fast, easy solution. This program is adaptable for everyone regardless of your age, current complaints, medical history, genetic make-up, economic situation, etc. All the barriers to achieving health in this book have been removed except for *your commitment*. No one can make you want to be a health nut. No one can make you exercise or eat well. At the end of the day, you still have a choice and you can choose to be healthy or unhealthy. As you go along in this process, remind yourself of that. "I have a choice," are the most empowering words you can give to yourself. The second we feel weak or even unworthy will lead the way to unmet expectations and disappointment. Free yourself from any shackles holding you back. You get to choose your own destiny. My greatest wish for you is to not be another statistic.

The advice in the following chapters is meant to be easy-to-follow. All you have to do is plug the information (all or some) from this book into your life and let that be your new normal. I've outlined 15 recipes (5 snack, 5 breakfast, 5 lunch/dinner) and 15 exercises to get you going. All are modifiable to your own liking and difficulty level. I've structured a plan, but you can also "choose your own ending," so to speak.

If you're reading along and you find yourself saying, I've done and tried everything and I've failed, then this is perfect for you. There is no such thing as failure when you're trying to turn your health around. Every step you take towards health, no matter how small and regardless of what the scale says, is a victory! Revel in every moment that you choose to be a healthier person and forget about those times that you felt weak. Every person has the potential to be a warrior: ambitious and fabulous! Do not let naysayers drag you down the rabbit hole of "your genes are working against you," or "you don't have the time," or "you've always been this way and you can't change" or any of the like. You are everything you need to be at this moment right now and you get to decide your fate. Will you choose sickness, dis-ease and death or will you choose vibrancy, sunshine and life?

Smile, baby. Today is your day!

Chapter 1:

The Facts and The Crisis

To honor full disclosure: I lived in Wisconsin. Wisconsin isn't the fattest state in the nation, but it certainly isn't the healthiest. We proudly declare that we consume more than 90% of the nation's brandy, can drink almost anyone under the table and have a serious love affair with cheese. I wish these things were exaggerations... but, alas, they are all truths. There is also an inherent pride or coolness in all the things we do that make us unhealthy. I find that to be especially true in young adults. Binge drinking, smoking, no savings, lack of sleep seem to be a rite of passage and maybe they are! But there are consequences when the young people of a country choose to carry those "young and dumb" habits into their adult lives. Their decisions can change the landscape of our country quickly.

Ready for some big numbers? Here are a few:

420,000

600,000

587,000

2,900,000,000,000

What do all these numbers mean? Let's take the 420,000. World War II was considered the deadliest war this world has ever known. It devastated countries, killed many innocent lives and leveled cities to dust. Four hundred and twenty thousand estimated Americans lost their lives in WWII. There are monuments erected to remember these brave souls. We celebrate and commemorate our veterans and they are given the highest esteem in our society. It is a reminder of the destruction of war and the value of peaceful times.

600,000 Americans will die THIS YEAR from heart disease alone.

An estimated **587,000** Americans will lose their battle with cancer THIS YEAR.

We spend **$2.9 trillion** on healthcare every year and that number continues to rise.

It has become the status quo to be sick, take medication and have surgery. The average young person in the U.S. takes 4 drugs, middle age takes 12 and the average person over the age of 65 takes 27 prescription medications! This would be acceptable if we were growing to be a healthier country by leaps and bounds, but that is not the case.

There is a time and place for drugs and surgery, and thank God there are people trained in cutting people open and administering prescriptions that save lives. There are times we need those things. If my leg is broken, I'm not going to a chiropractor. There is a doctor you go to when you are sick, so there should be a doctor you go to to maintain health. You need both! You need someone to advocate for your weight loss and be your coach. Some people need a guide on how to be healthier and maintain a level of wellness. Those doctors are naturopaths, chiropractors, homeopaths, acupuncturists and medical doctors too. It is also the responsibility of these wellness advisors to recognize when a person needs urgent and aggressive medical attention as well. It takes everyone cooperating and pushing towards a new paradigm in our society to make this country strong again.

Over 60% of the United States' population has weight to lose. That's the majority. Obesity is not just a matter of food choices it's lifestyle choices. Obesity, while it is a disease, can be managed safely and effectively without surgery and without drugs. Love yourself enough to be healthier! Strive for greatness. Maybe you feel like you don't have a pound to lose. Great! But being at your optimal weight will give your energy, have a more positive attitude, you might even sleep better and have an incredible sex drive! Don't you also want those things for yourself?

I can look around a room full of people and see those who are both healthier and sicker than me. For most of my life, that will be true. Someone will always be healthier and I can always find someone who is not as healthy as me. This way, I can say that my health is good (not excellent or poor). The problem with this way of thinking is that everyone else can do that too. What I mean is that if I were 40 pounds overweight, taking a few prescription drugs to help with symptoms of chronic illness, but did some walking every day, I could say the same thing. That my health is average and that "that guy over there" is way less healthy than me, so I'm still good.

We should stop comparing our health to those of other people. Compare you to you. Compare your health today to 10 years ago. What has changed? Were they good changes? So what if you made poor health choices when you were younger. Choose to act differently now!

On October 19, 2013, my son was born. Everyone told me he would change everything, and boy were they right! I was prepared for the sleepless nights, a weird and different version of my body and hormonal surges that sent me into fits of giggles and then tears moments later. What I wasn't prepared for was how I would view the world. The world was all of a sudden scarier. Before, the world was my oyster, any city was home and I felt on top of it all. I could make decisions in a moment with few consequences and no one else to consider.

Once that little being was put on my chest, the world was different. I became more nervous that the doors weren't locked at night or that my diet needed to be perfect for this little being to thrive. I became more concerned about what others were doing around my kid when before "It's your life" was my motto. I saw where healthcare was going. I see the obesity rates in children skyrocketing along with Type II diabetes and it scares me. If you have children and have been kept up at night worrying about their safety, you get it. But this is what keeps me up at night and why we need to change our behaviors now: What kind of world are we leaving for our kids?

Am I asking Max to take on the burdens of a nation who decided that being unhealthy was OK? This will be the first generation to not extend the life expectancy. I still cannot wrap my head around that.

As a parent of two now, this resonates so deeply with me and is the main motivator for why I do what I do. I will fight tirelessly to better the world my children live in and I'm asking you to do the same. You can choose to keep your kids active and moving. Kids need fresh air, exercise, free play and interaction with others! We are leaving behind a country that will be crippled with the inability to socially interact. Do not let the innocents shoulder the burden of a problem we created. Be the change, make a difference and choose health.

We are all in this together. It seems that everyone has a finger to point. Insurance companies, the patient, the doctor, the hospital and so on. Many people no longer have trusting relationships with their doctors and/or can't afford to see them anyway. $20,000 deductibles and mechanized doctor visits have become acceptable. The word 'doctor' can be translated to mean 'most learned one' or 'teacher' and they are! Doctors study intensely for a good majority of their lives to achieve a level of knowledge to share with others. Not all are good, that's true. But most are and are willing to help you in any way they can, but they also need to be reminded of the importance of asking the right questions. The process needs to change from, "Your tests came back and you have Diabetes, here's your Metformin," to "You have Diabetes, let's get your diet under control and start exercising." If your doctor isn't bringing that to the table, you can and should start the conversation! It does take a certain amount of pride swallowing on your end to admit there's a problem, but, like I said before, love yourself enough to be better.

I'll admit in my early years of practice I all too quickly pointed my finger at the medical community and said, "YOU! You are the problem and I hate you!" My mother said that with age comes wisdom and, what do you know, mama was right. There are no more fingers to point. No more scapegoats. We all have our roles to play and it is going to take all of our efforts to dig ourselves out of this tremendous sick hole we have dug. You may have made poor decisions in the past or went back on promises you made to yourself to be better. It's okay! Join me now on this journey and get back on your feet!

To shift your health, we must shift the paradigm.

You can be the change.

You can start a movement.

To be a healthier nation, we can no longer rely on drugs and surgery to aid us. We have to think that there is no miracle drug to come that can replace the benefits of a healthy diet and regular exercise. We were meant to move our bodies and eat foods that came from the Earth. Are you willing to make changes in your life? What would you be willing to sacrifice? Who are you changing for?

Chapter 2:

It's not your fault

Caveat: It's not ALL your fault. Companies spend billions of dollars marketing items for you to buy. The food industry, the health industry, the pharmaceutical industry, the whatever industry *have* to sell you their merchandise or they wouldn't be in business. Some of those companies advertise in the spirit of good intentions, but their goal at the end of the day is to sell you their products. Period.

The intensity and volume of ads is staggering. We, and our kids, are presented with thousands of targeted ads every day trying to convince us that this will make us happy, thin, wealthy, a good parent... Google and Facebook can even track the pattern of your clicks on a website to send you ads specific to what you've been searching for. The issue with this comes when we rely on the advertising or packaging of a product to determine the truth of that product. This is especially true in the food industry. "All Natural", "Fat-free", "Zero Calorie", "Cage free", are all phrases we've seen a thousand times. We assume those things should be healthier for us because it's on the label!

This type of advertising was not such a perverse issue 100 years ago. To understand why this is so huge, let's step back to the time of our earliest ancestors when there were times of feast and times of famine. Being eaten by wild boars was a real possibility and food was considered fast if it could outrun you. You ate nuts, seeds, fruits, vegetables and lean meats. There were no other options. There were no aisles or bright colored packages telling you what to eat. This lifestyle continued until the agricultural age when we started planting things and harvesting, and so on and so forth. It is just recently, in the last century that our diets have changed so dramatically that evolution cannot keep up with us.

Food is *everywhere*. Most corners house a Burger King or McDonald's, Golden Corral offering all-you-can-eat buffets on TV, radio and billboards. We are bombarded with food media. Some is good, most are bad. We are still equipped with caveman processes that are trying to take on space age food, chemicals and additives. Our bodies don't know what to do with it all.

The point of this field trip is to demonstrate that there are evolutionary traits that have been developing since the beginning of time, and for always, to dictate the processes our body needs to survive. We need to eat food to thrive. Our food is broken down in a very specific way. There's a symphony of chemicals and digestive movement. Every system in our body has been intelligently designed by time. One of many pearls of wisdom I gained from my father-in-law was "God didn't make a shitty product."

Your body is constantly trying to maintain balance. This balance, in the nerdy medical world, is called homeostasis. We are being bombarded with elements and stresses and chemicals and other things that throw our bodies out of homeostasis. Your body will adapt and deal with it until it can no longer adapt... this is when we start to see disease. A diagnosis is simply your body's way of telling you it's in turmoil. When you exhibit signs of Type II Diabetes, your body is telling you it's struggling. That it has been fighting for too long and can no longer deal with the stress and it is starting to sink. It's the same with high blood pressure, high cholesterol, depression, cancer and a long list of others. Don't be discouraged, though. There are still lots of ways to change this.

Let's go back to the cave man. We talked about feasts and famines. The cave man knew that before a famine s/he would need to seek out foods that were high in sugar and fat to pack on the pounds in order to survive. Our brain chemistry is designed to desire these foods because, back in the day, they were scarce but necessary for survival. That process didn't just go away when food became readily available at every corner. Evolution doesn't work that fast. *Your brain still wants you to seek out those foods to prepare for the inevitable famine.* What your brain doesn't know is that the famine for most never comes, so the extra calories taken in get stored efficiently as fat.

Not only is evolution working against you but so are the corporations who make food! Food has been designed to look, smell, feel and taste more delicious so that you, the consumer, will buy it. Most of the food being sold in the middle aisles of the grocery store isn't really food: it's food-like product. Flavor enhancers are used in most packaged items to give foods devoid of real nutrition a huge flavor punch. Artificial sweeteners are marketed as being sugar-free and healthier for you when in fact they excite your brain to a level of neurotoxicity. These things are made in a lab, not in nature. You are consuming a science experiment. It's a clever game this food industry is playing, but you can win!

Did you know that heart disease and Type II Diabetes can be reversed? It seems that once someone is put on a medication they need to be on it for life which may be necessary. Doctors understand the effectiveness of the status quo and how reluctant people are to change. It is sometimes easier to have a person take a pill every day than to advise them on a whole new life and trust them to follow through.

A main contributor to making a diagnosis is in the family history portion of a medical intake form. Your genetics do play a part in that they can make you more susceptible to certain diseases, but that's not the whole story.

Take a moment to picture a scenario: a family of four living in New York City. The parents are morbidly obese. The two kids are identical twins, have lived in the same house, ate the same food, inhaled similar toxins and have been exposed to the same chemicals. Twin A leaves the house and continues the habits his family taught him about eating poorly and having a sedentary lifestyle. Twin B leaves the house and joins a gym with a trainer, changes his entire diet and starts seeing a counselor to help him adapt to this new lifestyle. Who is less likely to have heart disease later in life? Who would be less likely to suffer from depression? Twin A or B? Identical DNA, and yet we all know the answer. What would happen if the twins were given up for adoption and put in homes that embraced the wellness lifestyle?

I ask these questions to challenge a very common thread that's being thrown around like it's law in our society: that genes control our health. Genetics only play a role, but our decisions and actions determine how those genes are expressed. Can a healthy diet, regular exercise and positive mental attitude ward off cancer? The research is pointing to yes!

The study of lifestyle decisions determining gene expression is called epigenetics. Those in this field will probably cringe at the next analogy. Think of each gene as contributing to a particular part of you: Your blue eyes, your blonde hair, your hitchhiker's thumb, your weight, etc. Now, imagine that some of those genes have an on/off switch. Your family history of chronic disease has an on/off switch that can change due to the environment your body lives in. When your doctor mentions family history, do not let that tip the scales on your decision to take a life altering medication. We do not put enough emphasis on the fact that prescription drugs, although super common, alter our chemistry and have dangerous side effects. Just because you can list 50 people who take a high blood pressure medication, doesn't mean that they're without risk. It's a big decision! Every alternative option should be explored before we change the processes that our body has taken millions of years to develop all because Grandpa had Diabetes.

Armed with knowledge, approach the doctor you chose to be in charge of keeping you well and ask questions. Is this right for me? What do you think? Is it worth a shot? *Will you help me?* The answers may surprise you.

Chapter: 3

Getting Started and Getting Your Head in the Game

The hardest part of any change is coping with its permanence. Sometimes we change for a short time and quickly change back to our original selves if the change isn't what we expected. There are habits we've created that become part of our identity and that we feel define us. How hard is it to change those things that we feel make us who we are?

I don't think anyone can argue that death is concretely permanent. Many of us have unfortunately become very familiar with death myself being amongst them. Kids I went to school with, grandparents, aunts, uncles, cousins, friends: I've known many who have left us before their time. My Uncle Tracy's passing was certainly the hardest loss I've faced. When my uncle died at age 46, a week before he was to marry his soul mate of 15 years, it was like someone knocked the wind out of me. It was incomprehensible to me. Maybe because he had a larger than life character that I never thought could be silenced. His sarcastic but well-meant euphemisms are still joked about. It was hard to imagine he wouldn't be posting his infamous TGIF Facebook posts anymore. That sounds so trite as I read it back to myself, but it's true. The permanence of death is so difficult and the simple fact that I had looked at my Facebook page for the last 10 years and now knew I was not going to see another interpretation of TGIF (Thinks Gigi is Fantastic, Thinks Gigi is Fun...) was hard to grasp.

While death is an extreme example, lifestyle changes can also be as absolute if you let them be. That is step #1. When choosing a different lifestyle, allow your choices to be permanent. Become familiar with their permanence in your life and use it to your advantage. Mourn your junk food and bad habits. Accept that you had some great times together, and then let them go. Your life is going to be different starting today. This may be a 90-day start-up, but it's a lifestyle overhaul that you must accept into your life, or your goals will be that much harder to achieve.

Try adopting all the labels that come with being healthy even if you're not into that kind of thing. Play with the idea of being an exercise junkie, a health food nut, a non-smoker. Imagine yourself being that person. Think about how you'll feel, what you'll say to other people, what you'll wear. Do not in the beginning stages remind yourself of how hard it's going to be. Imagining is half the fun, so don't focus on negativity right out of the gates! Imagine these things even if you don't believe them at first and the very idea makes you laugh. Just the act of thinking the way you want changes your chemistry. It's just science…

When you've been given a diagnosis from a doctor that label sticks with you, doesn't it? Hello. I have cancer. Hello. I'm depressed. Hello. I'm obese. You can lean on those labels to define you. They become your every thought, dictate your decisions and activities and can change your life instantly. If those labels stick, why can't others? Why shouldn't you use labels of your own design to enhance your self-confidence? If you can visualize yourself as a healthier person, you've already done a lot of the hard work. Any person who has lost a significant amount of weight will tell you that one of the hardest things was to realize that they were no longer the fat guy or girl. Their whole identity needed to change. If you do that from the start, you are light years ahead of everyone else and it doesn't cost you a dime!

In addition to visualizing, writing down your goals is crucial. People who physically write down their goals are 80% more likely to achieve them. And, again, it costs nothing. Don't be afraid to set lofty goals even if they seem unattainable right now. There are lots of coaches and experts who will tell you to set reasonable goals so that you won't get discouraged. My advice is to set your dream first and work backwards from there, setting reasonable goals as checkpoints. Write your goals as if they've already happened.

Like this:

I lost 100 pounds

I love to go to spin class

I run 5K's all the time

I'm an early riser (my sister just laughed out loud reading this one, I know it).

Use your goals as daily affirmations instead of reminders of how far you have to go. Achieving goals should be fun! Not daunting or disheartening. Most importantly when you are preparing to get your head in the game, know that you will face your demons. You will have moments of crazy, ugly crying, self-hatred and the overwhelming sense that you can't go on another minute. You will show weakness and cave in. You will not be perfect every day because no one is. Recognize those moments and acknowledge when they happen. Every road has bumps, and you will certainly have yours. Do not let bumps or detours be road blocks. I'm giving you permission now to have bad days and to be overwhelmed. You are allowed to do those things.

Health is a journey, not a destination and maybe you needed to make that pit stop along the way to really learn the right path for you. Try to see those moments of weakness as valuable learning tools and don't allow yourself to be beaten down with self-loathing. You will find that once you start giving your body the things that it needs, it's going to take care of you in a way you never thought possible. Once your mind and spirit start to connect with your physical body, you will be unstoppable, and what seems hard today will be a breeze in the future. You will be fearless. Trust in that and trust in you.

An important aspect of starting anything new is understanding why you are doing it. I think it is wonderful when people set goals like to lose 20 pounds before Spring Break. There's an attainable goal and a timeframe that is realistic. If you took that goal one step further, it makes all the difference in the world. "I'm losing 20 pounds before Spring Break because I want to feel confident wearing a bikini," and then share with yourself the plan on how to do it. Physically writing out a plan to achieve your goals will exponentially increase the likelihood of you achieving it. Attaching an emotion or a way you want to feel is like pouring gas on the fire! Plan for making big steps or baby steps towards your goal. Maybe you want to start slow and that's OK.

If your goal is connected to tackling a chronic condition, I would like to explain, in simple terms, how that condition affects the body. When you're given a diagnosis you are typically handed a brochure or print out on what that diagnosis is, how to treat it and a prescription to start taking. There are many physicians who do not go to the trouble of explaining what is actually happening inside your body simply because they are not allowed the time.

The following are the most common chronic illnesses/symptoms that people are suffering from hopefully explained in the easiest way.

Cancer

We'll start with the scariest. Getting a cancer diagnosis is like getting punched in the throat. Cancer is when your own cells from whatever tissue or organ (skin, breast, lung) grow uncontrollably. It can migrate and cause cancer in other areas. You can have breast tissue grow elsewhere in your body, which is called metastasis. The truth is, we are fighting cancer at all times. You have cancer right now... but your body keeps the cells from multiplying more than they need to. We are constantly turning over old cells and making new ones. There's a little chemical called tumor necrosis factor that causes cells to die before they get too large or too many. This is the guy that keeps you from getting cancer.

When a tumor (or a large group of cells replicating faster than they should) is found, doctors go in, remove it and then do radiation or chemotherapy which is the attempt to stop cell growth... all cell growth. The question: why did that group of cells suddenly decide after that many years to start multiplying and multiplying? The answer: Lots of reasons, all theories. Genetics play a role, but how

much of a role? The World Health Organization stated that nearly half of all cancers may be prevented with diet and exercise changes. Interesting, no?

Diabetes

There are 2 types of Diabetes mellitus, I and II. Type I is often diagnosed in childhood and can

also be called insulin-dependent. Go with me on this journey of physiology because this is one of the fastest growing diseases in the country and should be well understood by all.

The pancreas is this ugly little organ that sits close to the stomach and beginning part of the small intestine. It has many jobs, but its main job is to produce insulin. Insulin is a protein that acts like a taxi service for sugar. When you eat food, it gets broken down into chemicals and products, one of those being sugar/glucose. Once sugar is in the blood stream, it hails a cab. Insulin pulls over and picks up sugar who immediately says, "Take me to a cell. I'm in a hurry and need to make energy for this human," and insulin drives off to an energy-making cell and drops sugar off inside. With Type I Diabetes, there's a ton of sugar needing a ride, but no cabbies. The pancreas is not producing enough insulin. That is why they need to inject insulin in order to control their blood sugar.

Type II Diabetes is quite different. If you are Type II Diabetic, your cabbies are running wild! There are way too many. They're bumping into each other and wrecking storefronts and hitting pedestrians as they drop off sugar. Pretty soon, there is not enough room for the cabs to stop at the curb, so sugar gets stuck in gridlock traffic and blood sugar goes up uncontrollably. Insulin needs to be controlled and the receptors (storefronts/curbs) need to be repaired.

A common misconception is that once those insulin receptors are damaged, they can never be replaced and you will have to be on medication forever. New research is saying that that might not be the case. Changing your diet and adopting this 90-Day Plan will put you on the track to reversing that diagnosis. Be careful, though. Sugar isn't just in cookies and cake. When we eat bread, hot dog or

hamburger buns, pancakes, bagels, crackers, etc. they all get broken down as sugar in our bodies. They might not taste sweet in our mouths, but they taste sweet to our pancreas.

High Cholesterol

Eating lots of cholesterol will not necessarily give you high cholesterol. Eating a fat-free diet will not necessarily lower your cholesterol. Shocked? So was I.

We need cholesterol in your body to make important things like hormones, cell membranes, and it is a large contributor in the process of making energy for our bodies. It's really important and we can't just not have it. There is also good and bad cholesterol, although you need a balance of both to be healthy. LDL (low density lipoprotein) is bad, HDL (high density) is good. LDL's are sticky, gunky and get caught up in our vessels causing plaques and stiff vessels when in the presence of inflammation. The common treatment is the statin drug. Statins stop production of cholesterol in the liver which accounts for roughly 70% of all cholesterol production.

Fats are a necessary part of our diet, but some are better than others. Eating trans-fat, processed oils, fried foods will give you high bad cholesterol while olive oil, coconut oil and/or avocado oil will help maintain healthy cholesterol. Beyond fat consumption, the graph above shows that sugar is the main component to having high cholesterol. Compare fat-free anything to regular. Fat content goes down, but what goes up? SUGAR! They have to make it taste good or no one will buy it. When you eat excessive amounts of sugar and flour, after your blood sugar spikes and insulin is released to carry it away, that excessive insulin stimulates an enzyme with a very long name that tells the liver to start kicking out cholesterol. If you're on a statin, your liver is being told not to do that. Where does the sugar go? Back into the blood stream. Conclusion: if you continue to eat lots of sugar while on a statin, you will shortly find yourself with Type II Diabetes as well.

I'll never forget a story my dear friend, Dr. Scott Kurtti, told me. He was on a plane headed to New York to visit his son. On the way, he sat next to some big-wig cardiovascular surgeon and they got to chatting. This surgeon was published and highly respected in his community. Do you know what he told Dr. Kurtti? This is what he said: "If I could put everyone on a statin drug I would. It's the best thing to keep people healthy."

.... I'm sure this man is very smart and has nothing but the best of intentions for his patients, but it isn't as simple as putting everyone on a drug and calling it a day. There are devastating side effects to taking a statin for long periods of time: Muscle break down, chronic fatigue, chronic pain, headaches, sleep difficulties, all kinds of GI problems, memory loss, mental confusion and, of course, high blood sugar. I mean, they're right on the insert.

High Blood Pressure

Your body has a flow. Blood from the heart circulates around transporting stuff to the body and then goes back to the lungs and heart to recharge and then flows back out again. Our vessels on the way out expand and contract to pump and then blood slowly flows back via our veins. If somewhere along the line a vessel can't expand like it's supposed to or there's a road block to where the flow can't get through as fast, the pressure builds behind it = High Blood Pressure.

High blood pressure can also be caused by a normal response of our heart pumping more blood than usual faster through our system like in times when we're nervous, scared or angry. If you have in increase in the amount of blood in your body, like ladies when they're pregnant, you can also have times of high blood pressure. Most of the time, your nurse or doctor will tell you 2 numbers, a bottom and a top number. The top number is the pressure when your heart contracts to release blood to the rest of your body and the bottom number is the pressure when it's filling back up.

There are lots of treatments out there, but few address the real root of the issue: Why is there a road block in your system? Diuretics make the blood thinner so it flows easier around the road blocks, beta blockers slow your heart so blood has more time to get around the road blocks, ACE inhibitors, ARB's and calcium channel blockers relax your vessels so that more blood can fit around the road blocks. Am I missing something? Can heart disease be reversed? Can plaques be removed? Research says yes!

Depression

This is a tough one to explain simply because there are so, so many contributing factors to depression. We most commonly look to the chemicals serotonin, norepinephrine and dopamine as the main contributors to feeling happy or sad, but these alone cannot explain the complex interconnectivity of our body systems when someone is depressed. Emotions are not well understood. To be sure, chemicals are involved and an imbalance is assumed.

Depression can be felt all over, but it is mostly felt in the brain, specifically the amygdala, the thalamus and the hippocampus. The amygdala and hippocampus are part of our emotional center called the Limbic System. Here's the system: the thalamus is like the secretary of the brain. It receives impulses from all over and then sends it to whichever part of the brain that particular impulse needs to land. The hippocampus and amygdala talk back and forth at the water cooler. The hippocampus remembers things that have happened to you, good and bad, and then relays those memories to the amygdala who decides whether that memory should elicit anger, happiness, arousal, sympathy and so on. These messages are sent to our hormone system and a million other centers to respond the way our brain decides. Different chemicals are released when we feel sad versus when we are elated.

Anti-depressants dampen the whole system. They control the release and exit of those 3 chemicals to create different messages that are sent to the brain. Research shows that a healthy diet and regular exercise are more effective at treating depression than anti-depressants. With something so complex and still somewhat elusive, is it ethical to simply take a drug that alters the way your brain communicates with itself and the rest of your body? Maybe. What else could be affected by changing these processes? Would you be willing to sacrifice feeling happy to not feel sad? Would you be willing to try something different?

Arthritis

Arthritis is just part of a chiropractor's life. We see it all day long, on x-ray, on the medication
list and hearing about people's achin' backs. Arthritis is a general term for breakdown of a joint. Any joint can be affected. There are lots of types, but they boil down to 2 different families of arthritis: the non-inflammatory and the inflammatory. Non-inflammatory is the wear-and-tear, hard-on-your-body type when the cartilage deteriorates over time or due to unusual amounts of stress put on that joint. It can also be caused or quickened by nutritional deficiency or surgical procedures.

Inflammatory arthritis doesn't just affect joints. For example, enteric arthritis is secondary to Crohn's disease, ulcerative colitis and inflammatory bowel disease. There are autoimmune diseases that attack joints, infections that leave a joint weakened and susceptible and a myriad of other causes. The tricky part is that arthritis might not necessarily cause pain or be the cause of your pain. When you see extensive arthritis on an x-ray, the true determinant as to whether that arthritis will cause pain or not is how deconditioned that individual is. If a person has a healthy diet and is relatively active, the arthritis could go unnoticed forever and never cause any issues. On the other hand, if a person has poor muscle strength, inflammatory diet and leads a sedentary life, they are more likely to suffer from pain.

I'll typically hear patients proclaim that it's their age that plagues them, which I suppose it is to a small degree. Don't be fooled, just because you're older than some does not mean arthritis has to be part of your life. It is not inevitable. There is little to no research suggesting that regular chiropractic care prevents or reduces the amount of arthritis you develop. But time and time again, we compare the x-rays of someone 70+ years old who has been getting adjusted forever to someone in the 30's who doesn't believe in chiropractic and the findings are astounding! Does that shock you? I hope it does.

Obesity

The newcomer to the table: obesity. Since the 1970's, obesity has been on the rise and is linked to every disease process listed above and many, many others. Simply put, if you consume more calories than what your body needs, those extra calories get stored as fat. We spoke of the cave man earlier and how your body was designed to go through feasts and famines. The reality is that we are consuming more calories than ever that are devoid of any real nutritive value. We're overeating, yet starving.

Perhaps what is lesser known is that you can lose fat, but you cannot change the number of fat cells in your body. Unfortunately, once you have created a fat cell, it is with you forever. There is some debate as to whether certain programs or supplements can in fact kill fat cells, but nothing concrete or safe has come to the surface. When a cell becomes overloaded with storage, the body creates more fat cells to deal with the burden. Diet and exercise will shrink the size of the cell, but it cannot be eliminated entirely. That is part of the reason why it is so easy to gain weight back. If you have been overweight in the past, you have the same number of fat cells they are just smaller than they used to be.

Like depression, this is not a simple condition. There are addictions, body issues and self-esteem issues that must be addressed along with caloric intake, nutrient levels and portion size. You must recognize the whole picture before fixing the minutia.

In closing, I'll say this: it will take a steady routine and habitual planning to achieve health. We think too often that it is a matter of inner strength that some people have and others don't that achieves goals. "I am a weak person therefore I can't do this." We look at others who accomplish things easily and think, "Look how determined they are. They're so disciplined. I could never do that." The difference between someone who achieves and someone who thinks they have failed is a decision to do either.

I do not believe in will power. I think it's a made-up thing. Taking this journey will require purposeful action steps every day for *yourself.* Achieve your goals because they are only yours to achieve. The only person out there thinking you are weak is you. You might not have a routine now, but you will. You might not understand your own strength at this moment, but you will. You might not have it all figured out right now, but you will. Take a chance and leap!

Chapter 4:

Nutrition

Think of your body as this incredible machine. You really don't have to do any of the hardwiring or construction. It was given to you pre-fab. All you have to do is give it regular maintenance like changing the oil, rotating the tires and refilling the fluids. Sounds easy, right? It certainly can be. The hard part is when your machine gets neglected or the wrong things and parts are used for years and years. You now have to pay a mechanic thousands of dollars because you didn't change the oil for 50,000 miles.

I see this a lot in the chiropractic world. Maybe someone got in a few fender benders, didn't exercise and sat at a desk all day. One day, their back will go out and s/he will come to their friendly chiropractor to fix it and are in disbelief when I say it's going to take 3-6 months to get them healed and stable. If you abuse yourself for years, please do not expect a quick fix. The same goes for every aspect of your health.

Are you due for an oil change? If your body is like a car, think of food as the fuel and fluids necessary. What would happen if you put water in your gas tank or eggs in your radiator? Other than something foul smelling, your car wouldn't run very well or for very long.

Your diet and nutrition are vital. In the United States, we don't think of food as fuel. We consider food as something we put in our bodies because we're hungry or stressed or bored or trying to fill some other void. But food is simply food. It is inanimate. It cannot love you and we cannot feel anything for food, or we shouldn't. We are meant to consume food for the sole purpose of nourishing our bodies. Food has no other biological function other than to keep us alive.

Do you have comfort foods? When you're feeling sad you have go-to meals that give you the warm fuzzies? Step back for a moment and realize how incredibly weird that is. My friend's mother was advised by her physician to cut back on the sweets. Her response was, "I would rather die than give up my peanut M&M's..." And whether or not she truly feels that way or not, the simple exclamation is enough to cause an eyebrow to raise. *My* M&M's... Unless you're a black widow, we should not have feelings towards our food. Now, eating food should also be enjoyable! If we start to hate eating food... that's a problem as well. Start a new love affair. Cut the ties between you and McDonald's and go steady with the hot new spring mix salad or sautéed kale. Try foods you think you won't like in different ways with different seasonings. The back pages of this book are chock-full of recipes that are simple, easy and incredibly nutritious. Super foods, so to speak.

Your entire bodily chemistry changes when the diet is changed from junk to whole foods. A majority of packaged foods (anything in a can, box or bag) have been altered or preserved using chemicals that are not known to nature. Our brains light up like Christmas trees in our pleasure centers when we eat foods high in sugar, fat, salt, etc. When flavor enhancers (like MSG, aspartame, sorbitol) are used, our brains get so excited they think you're high. Literally. The same areas that fire up when you take drugs ignite when you eat those things. You have been deceived! It is not your bad habits that make you crave foods. They are **designed** to make you love them.

As mentioned before, it is very easy to get caught up in the outside packaging that promises fat-free or diet something. It sounds healthier than the regular product so the package should deliver on its promise. While things that are diet or fat-free have fewer calories and fats which might seem healthier in the beginning, they are also filled with sugar, sodium and chemicals. That combination of ingredients changes the way our bodies recognize when we're full: satiation signals.

Take diet soda as an example. There are fewer calories and maybe less sugar, so how do they make it taste good? They add aspartame or other artificial sweeteners. When consumed your brain lights up saying that it really likes what it's getting, but forgets to tell your stomach about the consumption. You will feel hungry *sooner and faster* than if you drank a regular soda. Hunger triggers you to eat more calories thus more weight gained despite the diet label.

As a consumer, there are a lot of options if you would like to diet. You can almost cherry pick a diet to accommodate whatever food you feel like you "couldn't live without." I could ask 10 people on the street what a healthy diet looks like and they could all say something different. There's no standard.

What does a healthy diet look like? It used to be very simple and still is simple in other countries. We are exposed to a crazy amount of advertising promising an endless list of dreams. It's hard to know what is just clever marketing and what is actually good and healthy. It's difficult as a consumer to piece apart the good information from the not-so-good.

Whenever someone asks for advice on how and what to eat, I say this: *Eat what your ancestors ate.* Not everything from the past should be taken as law (lack of hygiene and frontal lobotomies being at the top of the list), but where our food comes from and what are plates look like should not be changing all that dramatically from one era to the next. Evolution hasn't changed us so much to adapt to a laundry list of chemicals and alterations being added to our food. There are common sense decisions you already know to be true. But the bottom line is *I cannot make*

you buy food, I cannot make you cook it and I certainly cannot make you eat it. You are the sole contributor to what goes into your body. You have ultimate control. Try to experiment and find foods that you love, like and would be willing to tolerate because they are just so nutritious and can't not eat them. Don't force yourself to eat foods you hate. You'll end up hating cooking and eating, and what fun is that?

Back to the question at hand: What does a healthy diet look like? It looks like this:

60% fruits and vegetables

25% protein source

5% healthy fats and oils

10%.... everything else (dairy, processed foods, breads...)

These percentages are somewhat flexible depending on your activity level. If you are an elite athlete, pregnant, or nursing your protein requirement may be closer to 30-35%. The take home message is that ***most of your plate should be fruits and vegetables!*** Those 2 groups contain the majority of vitamins and minerals required to keep our machines healthy and running properly.

There are 2 common misconceptions when considering eliminating dairy and wheat. Those concerns are where will I get calcium from and don't I need grains for fiber? Did you know that our bodies really don't require grains? Our bodies *do* require carbohydrates and fiber, which can be found in grains as well as a thousand other things. 130 grams daily is recommended and 25-38 g of that should be fiber. There are approximately 33 grams in one medium sweet potato, one cup of raw corn has approximately 27 grams and one regular potato and a cup of broccoli has 32 grams. Filling your plate with vegetables will get you your daily requirement and won't spike your blood sugar. Dairy is a source of calcium, but it's not the only one. Green leafy vegetables (kale, bok choy, collard greens), broccoli, figs, oranges, sardines, salmon, white beans, okra and almonds are all incredible sources, just to name a few.

Now, how to get those nutritious things on your plate? The odious task of grocery shopping. A good rule of thumb is to shop the perimeter of the grocery store and avoid the center aisles. The outer perimeter usually consists of produce, the deli, butcher, eggs, frozen veggies and meats... Packaged, processed and mostly inedible foods are kept in the middle aisles. Avoid at all costs! It is true that you cannot *only* shop the perimeter. I drink coffee and tea and those things are found in the middle aisles. I also enjoy making hummus, which requires garbanzo beans, tahini and olive oil that can only be found in the middle aisles.

The point is, sure, sometimes you have to venture into the dark precipices of the middle aisles, but a majority of your grocery shopping should be done at the perimeter. My route is this: I head to produce first and fill up my cart with the good stuff, head to the butcher and fill it with wild caught fish and organic lean meats, head around to the cheese and yogurt aisle and then go through the middle for the things I missed. I do not go down every middle aisle, only the ones that contain the stuff on my list.

Budget is a very important consideration. Most of us live within a budget and that goes for food expenditures as well. Sometimes we sacrifice on good food because the alternative is cheaper. I understand completely. I won't lie to you and tell you that it is less expensive to eat healthy. It isn't true. It does cost more to eat well, but not as much as you think. I have found that meal planning and weekly trips to the grocer are vital to staying on a budget. Plan your meals starting with some at the back of this book. You'll soon find your favorites and stock up on bulk items for recipes that are sure-fire winners. I can typically get food for a family of 4 for 1-2 weeks in 45 minutes and spend about $100. Also, consider bulk buying, farmer's markets and local discount grocers.

Your first grocery bill is going to shock and amaze you. Don't fret. It's just like when you move into a new house and you have to buy things like mustard and what not. Get the essentials and shopping becomes cheaper. Also, consider that once you cut out the garbage food and fill your cart with produce, it levels the playing field a bit as well. And what better investment is there than *you?!* None. Invest in good food. It's amazing what people will spend on things that are so meaningless and damaging to their wellbeing and yet skimp on one of the most important contributors to your health. Could you sacrifice 1 pack of cigarettes a week in order to buy a whole bag of apples? Could you brew your own coffee instead of buying Starbucks to find some extra cash for grass-fed beef? It's a decision, but where you spend your dollars is important. You tell your money where to go!

A quick word on food labels: what is the purpose of checking food labels? Some would like an idea of calorie content, fats, sugar amounts, etc. The ingredient list can also be important to some. A simpler way to shop is to buy foods that don't have labels. I'm not into calorie counting, restricting calories, checking labels, etc. First, it takes way too long to shop that way and I don't have time for that kind of research. Second, labeling is not of the highest standard in the United States anyway and is not a clear representation of what's actually in the product. Instead of checking labels, buy foods that don't have labels. It's very hard to go wrong with that technique. Unless you have severe allergies to certain ingredients, skip the reading.

Many people are concerned about calories. How many calories are too many or not enough? What is a calorie anyway? By definition, a calorie is a way to measure energy. There are small calories and large calories. The large calories are what are on the food label. There are 1,000 small calories in a big one. The scientific definition is the amount of energy it takes to bring 1 kilogram of water to 1 degree Celsius. The more calories in an item, the more energy it takes to burn.

The average adult should consume about 2,000 Calories in a day. This is adjusted for activity level, medical history, height and weight, so that someone who is 5' and 100 pounds would not require the same energy as a 6'4" 300-pound farm boy to function. Here's the problem: calorie counting has become very marketable. Those 100 calorie snacks might be low in calories, but they are loaded with sugar, processed ingredients and a slurry of other things. I can eat a 2,000 calorie diet in one meal at the Golden Corral. The *amount* of calories isn't as important as *where those calories come from and how/when they're being ingested.* Now someone who is 400 pounds and eats 10,000 calories will have to restrict his/her caloric intake, but not to 2,000 calories. Remember what a calorie is. It's energy!

Think of your metabolism like a furnace. The hotter the fire, the more wood you burn, right? Reducing your calories when you're working out or trying to boost your metabolism is like trying to build a fire with no wood. Feed your fire with good, wholesome food, listen to what your body is telling you and proceed from there.

Remember that you are a machine: A highly intelligent and adaptable machine. If you are eating 10,000 calories a day, your machine is accustomed to receiving that many calories. If you suddenly started eating 2,000 calories, your body will go into starvation mode and store all the food you eat as fat, even though you might have plenty to spare.

When someone tells me that they are intensely working out 4-5 days a week, getting enough sleep and watching their portions but they're gaining weight instead of losing, I ask what their diet looks like. Mind you, you will add muscle, which will up the scale, but if you're obese and doing this routine and still gaining weight, something's up. They usually answer with: nothing for breakfast (or coffee), a few snacks, a salad for lunch and a portion-controlled dinner. That is not enough to sustain your activity level! That is why calorie counting is not the most effective way to lose weight and gain energy.

I went to a seminar several years ago taught by Dr. David Seaman. The seminar was called Clinical Nutrition and was supposed to give us a fail-proof nutritional system that any patient could do and that we could implement in our offices that Monday morning. I had lots of paper and an extra pen to take down the massive amount of notes I was expecting. I thought to myself "how could we possibly learn everything we need to know about every chronic disease to give that specific of a nutrition plan in 8 hours." Silly me.

Dr. Seaman is a tall, lanky and sarcastic man with a wide smile and snarky personality. He approached the speaker's podium and went into his introduction. With pen poised, I anxiously awaited his protocols. After several snide comments directed towards the medical community, he took off his glasses and said this:

"If you're sitting there waiting for some fancy cook book recipe to cure diabetes or heart disease with nutrition and supplements, you came to the wrong frickin' seminar."

Well, shit.

"I'm not going to waste the next 8 hours of your time, so this is the protocol you should tell every one of your patients come Monday: ***Eat more vegetables***!"

This is not what I wanted to hear. I was looking for a recipe. I wanted the cookbook. I brought pages to write on! But he was so right, and that day changed my whole view on nutrition. Nutrition is simple and, as a country, we simply need to eat more vegetables. Will red yeast rice lower your cholesterol? Probably. But so will eating more vegetables. Will white willow bark help with pain? Maybe, but so will an anti-inflammatory, vegetable-rich diet.

"Let food be thy medicine..." Hippocrates (the father of medicine)

I believe there is a place for supplements and herbs, but they should be used only as building blocks to support a solid, foundational diet. There needs to be a plug-and-play plan that anyone can insert into their lives and see results. A plan effective for the person who has Diabetes or a relatively fit person wanting to bring their health to the next level or even the working single mom who has maybe 10 minutes to prepare a meal for her family that accommodates her and their nutritional needs.

At the end of the day, you have to do what is right for you and your family. If you have picky eaters at home, get them involved in the shopping experience. Let them pick out dinner that night. Help them search for recipes in books and online. Go ahead and take a quick peak (if you haven't already) at the recipes in the back. They all take less than 30 minutes to make, are nutritious and have names that are kid-friendly. I am very fortunate to not have any picky eaters in my house, but I feel for those moms and dads who do.

It is so important that your children understand what a good meal is. You are the parent and you are responsible for their little machines. Convenience should not outweigh nutritive value. How can we expect a child to learn like a healthy kid, play like a healthy kid, maintain a healthy weight, think positively, socialize, relax or live a long, fulfilled life if we don't provide them with the nutrients and vitamins to do so? What if your child is not meeting their full potential because their brains are not getting the nutrients it needs to think clear? What if their little bodies are so full of processed food-like product and sugars that it goes haywire? Of course, there are always birthday parties and holidays that derail a healthy regime, but when your child's entire diet consists of "treats" you're robbing them of their potential. You're taking away their shot at good health. You are simply waiting for them to be sick. If you choose not to change your own diet or maybe can't afford to do it all, at least feed your kids a proper diet. They will eventually be the ones taking care of us and leading this country. We need them to understand what healthy means. There is nothing more important than showing your child love and feeding them the good stuff. And after doting upon your children's great health, give yourself a pat on the back and get started on your own!

Chapter 5:

Exercise

There are many excuses out there to not exercise. I know, because I've used many of them myself. I have not always been the most active person. I was not a high school athlete, I didn't touch a weight machine voluntarily until I was a junior in my undergraduate studies and I smoked a pack a day for 6 years. Not the pinnacle of health. To this day I use the same excuses to justify to myself that I don't have the energy or the money or the time to enjoy some exercise. Exercise should be just that: Enjoyable! It's hard to begin a new exercise routine and if you hate doing it, what's the motivation to keep going?

My sister is one of my favorite people. She makes me laugh all the time and has this larger than life personality. She's always been a bit of a ham... an understatement for sure. She, unfortunately, has some health issues I won't go into great detail about, but needless to say she has never been able to establish a decent diet, maintain a regular exercise schedule and she leads a very high strung, emotional and stressful life. When I tell her that exercise has been shown to be more effective at treating depression than anti-depressant medications she has a long list of reasons why it won't work for her. Her body is different and reacts differently to exercise whether it be the lack of the runner's high or the feeling of accomplishment. She really hates exercising. Before she even gets going, she feels like she's failed.

If you started every morning thinking "This day is going to suck." Guess what will happen... Your days will suck. If you start every workout saying, "I am going to hate this," you probably will. The opposite is true as well. If you have spent your whole life thinking you are not a morning person, even if you have "proof" that you hate getting up early, start thinking and truly believing that you love getting up in the morning. You might be met with resistance when you do wake up early and you feel crappy, but overtime, the constant affirmation will retrain the way you think about that part of you.

Your body likes habits, and so does your mind. Fill your brain with positive affirmations and mental habits. One of my favorite things to do in the morning when I'm in the shower is to think of 3 things that I am grateful for. Just holding on to those 3 things throughout my day cushions my attitude if something bad happens. If you have a tough workout and you feel like you might vomit or get really sore the next day, just think: I'm sore because I built strength and I appreciate that my muscles function to allow me to do this. Or it was hard this time, but it will be easier next time. Mentally prepare for setbacks, but don't expect them to happen!

I thought that the first time I went to CrossFit it would be horrible. I resisted for a long time after seeing how hardcore everyone was screaming and hollering in triumph as they threw the barbell above their heads with some ungodly amount of weight attached to it. "That won't be me," I'd say to myself. But I went anyway. And the first time *was* horrible. I couldn't walk for days I was so sore. I went a second and a third time each time thinking this was my last because it was too intense for me. I thought of every excuse in the book including my small stature, but I went anyway. I changed my thinking from "This is going to be awful" to "I'm going to do my best." While CrossFit continues to be a struggle, which challenges me to the furthest extent, it is easier. Even as I write this, when I know I should be going at least 2-3 times a week but find time for 1-2 times a month, it's easier. I'm not an elite athlete, but I can pretend to be one, even if it's only in my mind. I'll be met with resistance when people lift heavier than me or can beat my time in a workout, but I'm happy with me and that feels great.

I believe there are some common misconceptions about exercise. The first myth being that you have to feel miserable and want to die during it to show that you're accomplishing something. Exercise should be vigorous, but it should also be enjoyable. Mihaly Csikszentmihalyi, a noted psychologist, studies and writes about "Flow". Flow is the term used to describe an activity that one does not do because it is hard or stressful, but because it is easy and creates sincere happiness when performed. You can experience Flow at almost any time. Flow is effortless and fun. For me, my flow is yoga. I've always had a knack for it and it doesn't require much thought for me to practice for a few minutes every day. It's my stress relief that just happens to also be exercise.

What's your flow? What's something that's easy for you to do that makes you genuinely happy? Take something that you love and try to incorporate it into an exercise routine. You might not be lucky enough to have your Flow be exercise. Perhaps you like to play the piano. Hold a squat against the wall while you play for a certain amount of time with the piano in front of you. Be novel! Be creative! I think many people get caught up in only doing the elliptical machine or a treadmill for 30 minutes because it's easy and takes little to no experience to operate. If that's your thing that's really great! If that's your flow, go with it! But do it because you love it, not because it's the only thing you know how to do. Most gyms have personnel that will help you use equipment if you ask.

Another point I will make is that you must change it up! Do you remember homeostasis? Your body is constantly trying to bring you to a point of balance and that holds true for exercise as well. You will adapt to whatever workout you are doing, your muscles will get bored and the gains you saw in the beginning will diminish. This is a common complaint amongst those who are trying to lose some poundage. When you start a program, it's completely new to your body, so your body releases fluids, build muscles, burns fat to return you to homeostasis. It will get the hang of your routine fairly quickly (within 3-4 weeks) so the same 30 minutes you powered through on the elliptical last month is old news to your body now. You will become more efficient at burning calories. If you surprise your body with some light weight lifting or interval cardio training or some Pilates, it will be thrown out of balance and will have to burn fat, build muscle and increase your metabolism to keep up with you. You can use homeostasis to your advantage!

Cardiovascular work is great and you will certainly see some results with just that, but I encourage everyone to try some varied functional workouts. There are a lot of studios and gyms out there who offer free classes. Try something new. It might be terrifying and you might feel embarrassed, but it's OK to get out of your comfort zone every now and again. At-home videos are a great first step. I'll say that when I'm in a class with a group of people versus by myself at home, I work harder, I move better, I'm more focused and I feel a part of a community, which is essential to maintain a healthy lifestyle. If you want to achieve true strength and endurance in your body, this type of exercise is vital. Lifting weights can be super intimidating especially when you see these muscly hulks putting up crazy amounts of weight. Start with 5 pounds, even 2.5 pounds if you'd like, and do some simple lifts for 5 repetitions each side and then see how you feel.

Always try to use free weights. Some weight machines that use pulleys or bars allow one side to dominate the other. For example, say you have an overdeveloped right side just from being right-hand dominant. Would you want to encourage that right side to continue to be stronger? Probably not. When you push the bars away from you, the weight mechanism is connected to the other side, there is no independent motion coming from both sides. Technically, you could do a chest press this way with one hand. Using free weights also adds a balance component. The machine is a controlled lift, whereas you have to create the control when you lift free weights. Try to buddy up though. We wouldn't want to have any accidents.

With that being said, I understand the aversion to fitness clubs and will hopefully guide you through exercises that you can easily do at-home, at the gym, on vacation and pretty much anywhere else you can find a little space. I prefer to work out with a group and visit a CrossFit gym regularly, but I'm in it for the socialization and community. The idea is to elevate your heart rate for at least 20 minutes, incorporate some strength training if you're ready and address flexibility issues. It can all be done in 30 minutes. I'll warn you now: if you are one those who will only do the exercises you like... find a partner or a support group to work out with even if it's simply a group of girls/guys coming to your house and getting your sweat on for 20 minutes. If you only do the things you like, you might not see the gains you expect.

As a yoga instructor, I have had to adapt poses and exercises for all walks of life. There was an elderly woman I was coaching one-on-one. She was incredibly strong (sometimes more of mind than body), but lacked flexibility and stamina, so we had to accommodate her extensively. It opened my eyes to a problem that I know many people have: that there are few exercises that people with mobility issues can perform on their own without assistance. If those people are living on a budget or lack health insurance, it would be difficult for them to hire a trainer or physical therapist/nurse to assist them in exercising.

The exercises I outline here can be advanced, modified and made easier so that any person can perform them, even those confined to a wheelchair. In this chapter, I've simply listed the exercises with pictures. The number of repetitions, sets and time allotments are entirely up to you and your abilities. I am not much of a planner and I don't like people telling me what to do, so if you would like to make your own schedule, that's cool, but stick to it!

Form is also incredibly important. If you feel pain when you're doing a particular exercise, you might need someone to watch you who knows the correct form to prevent you from injuring yourself. Try doing each exercise in slow motion and in front of a family member/friend/mirror to ensure proper form. There is no point in exercising if you hurt yourself and are out of commission for the next 4-6 weeks while you heal. You also wouldn't want to learn the wrong way to do something. Take things at your own pace. You have lots of time to achieve your goals even if you have a deadline like a wedding or vacation. You cannot force things into your body that don't want to be there. No pain, no gain has no place here. Be attentive to what your body needs. It's talking, are you listening?

You will also notice that these exercises are chiropractic friendly meaning they will not produce added pressure to your spine when done correctly. Exercising should be somewhat uncomfortable especially if it's new to you, but you should not be in excruciating pain. If you are, you're doing too much and you need to return to the more conservative exercise options. Note also that this isn't an exhaustive list. Swimming, cycling and rowing are all low impact sports that also give our hearts a work out that will allow you to advance when you are ready.

No time, no money, people will judge me, people will look at me, I don't know how to exercise, it hurts to exercise, I don't like exercising. There are lots of ways to talk yourself out of something. You might even fess up to being scared or intimidated. It's OK to feel a little trapped and without answers. My goal is to unlock hidden potential and for you to face your fears despite your efforts to let them control you. I'll bet you can do more than you think. You will surprise yourself on this journey maybe in a good way or maybe in a not so good way. Like I said before, I cannot make you do things and I cannot work out for you. You are the only one who can find the motivation to go for a walk or ask for help. You are the only one who can do that. If you are waiting for someone to do it for you, you will be waiting forever. There's no time to waste! Your body is craving it!

Chapter 6:

The 90-Day Plan

You are ready for this. You have been waiting for a program that's right for you and this is it! You have everything you need in your body right now to achieve great health. It may seem so far away, light years away, but look at tomorrow and use every day to learn and adapt. Every day, every moment you decide to take a healthier path, you're closer to that healthy person you hold in your mind. There are no backward steps, there are no cheat days, there are no bad days or I-hate-myself days, there is no point system. You are you, and you are simply spectacular. Let's begin:

There are two roads you can take: the hardcore road or the easin' into it road. I want to give you options. As a writer, you tend to be biased in your recommendations because you only know what *you* would do. I'm an "all in" personality. Some might not be. Decide which one you are and follow these steps accordingly.

The "All In" Road

Whenever I decide I want to boost my spirits or increase my energy, I start a detoxification program. There are lots of these out there like footbaths, supplement packages, etc. I'm one to err on the more natural side and I follow a food-guided detox, which I will share with you. It's very simple. Here we go:

The first 7 days

Eat this:

Fruits

Vegetables

Nuts

Seeds

Pure spices

Healthy oils

Coconut, olive (for dressings), grapeseed (for sautéing/baking/grilling)

Honey for sweetener

Water

Don't eat this:

Everything else

Sound crazy? It's not. There are many researchers out there who attest to the value of fasting for several days to cleanse. Think of it as flushing your radiator fluid.... Terrible imaging. Think of detoxing as hitting control + alt + delete on your body (better). Flushing out all the crap that has been locked away in your cells and starting fresh with whole foods. Juicing is a quick and easy way to get all of our daily nutrients into an easy-to-consume drink. You don't get the same fiber when you juice, but the first 7 days are all about taking it easy and that goes for your digestion as well. Juice takes little energy to digest, but packs a huge nutrient punch. You are nourishing your body to the very core of your cells.

Notice the list of acceptable foods in the first 3 days does not include grains, meat, dairy or processed foods of any kind. I promise you will be okay. Those things take a lot of energy to digest. The point of a detox is to utilize the least amount of energy for digestion to give your body a break.

It's only a week, but the effects can last a lifetime. It is a short amount of time to sacrifice those indulgences for the betterment of YOU. You will certainly face your demons in those 7 days. Your addictions will absolutely rear their ugly heads and you may be faced with monsters you've never seen before. You might feel like a crackhead going through withdrawal symptoms (food can be addictive, yes or yes?). To the contrary, you might feel revitalized, vibrant, energized, awake, alert, *ALIVE*. Your body is completely unknown to me, but you are its expert. Relish the moments where you feel weak and push past to a healthier, stronger you. It's OK to have moments of weakness. You are being programmed to fall in love with sugar, fat and salt. It is in your DNA to do so. It's OK to that you love these things. It is not OK to be a slave to them. Be stronger than the sweets you consume. Be stronger than the bag a potato chips that threaten your livelihood. You are in control and you decide what your hands bring to your mouth.

The "Easing Into It" Road

Reading through other lifestyle books, I find that some can be fairly negative. The restrictions are pretty wild and if you don't respond well to plans or strict guidelines, failure is somewhat assured. You end up hating a diet and maybe yourself because you're cheating too often or not following the rules. The guidelines outlined here in this less aggressive lifestyle plan are simply that: guidelines.

Instead of diving into a regimented program that cuts out some of the things you most adore, let's try a different approach. Instead of eliminating and restricting, let's simply add things we know that are good for us and take it from there.

The First 21 Days

Add These:

1. Eat a fruit or vegetable before you eat anything else

This goes for snack time too! Have lots of cut up fruits and veggies on hand. Even if you eat one celery stick before a Double Whopper with cheese, that's a win, friend! You will find that once you start choosing healthier things before you eat junk, your body will recognize that as a habit and start to expect the good stuff. Eventually, you won't crave the junk! You can eat whatever you want, but have a fruit or vegetable before it enters your mouth.

2. **Drink half your body weight in fluid ounces of water**

   It doesn't really matter at what time you drink your water at this point, just shoot for drinking lots of it. Proper hydration can change your mood, decrease muscle spasm, lessen hunger triggers and make you feel more alert! To note: water means water. Water doesn't mean fluids. Beer, soda, coffee... those don't count! You can still drink those things in addition to the recommended amount of water.

3. **Add a protein source to your breakfast**

   Eating like a king for breakfast gets your day started on the right foot. Protein is a sustainable energy source. Eggs, greek yogurt, nuts, bacon! I think the meats for breakfast have been demonized. While they do take a large amount of energy to digest, you also gain a significant amount of energy to carry you through the day. If you're not much of a cook, protein powders (I suggest pea protein) are out there and are easy to throw into some milk/water/juice and slug on your way out the door.

   And that's it! There are your first seven days outlined. Simple, right? Whether you're diving right into a detox plan or meandering your way through to see how your body responds, you're off to a great start! If you're going through the detox and are struggling, check out the easing into it road and start there. Instead of getting overwhelmed, try something different.

NOTE: You shouldn't start a heavy workout routine during these days. Try to drink lots of water and take a peek at some of the breathing exercises outlined in Chapter 5. Work on getting your head in the game and focusing on you. Confront fears and expectations. Journal. Take the first 7 seven days to establish goals as we outlined in Chapter 2.

For you who are going "All in", here is what the second week looks like for you:

Add these things:

Wild Rice, Brown Rice

Quinoa, steel-cut oats, millet

Beans, lentils, legumes

If you're easing into things, focus on every meal containing *at least* 50% fruits and vegetables. Fill your plate with a variety of colors, flavors, new foods that you would usually pass by in the store. If you're curious about an ingredient, use allrecipes.com or the Food Network app to look for new recipes. Most importantly, HAVE FUN exploring a new palette. We can very easily fall back on meals and flavors that we know we like. Explore new tastes. Some things you'll love and adopt into a new routine. Others you will hate and never eat again. You'll never know until you try!

The third week for you hardcore individuals looks like this:

Add these things:

Eggs

Lean meats (fish, organ meats, wild game)

Greek yogurt, kefir, hard cheeses

Now that we're introducing more and more things, you'll start to notice what agrees with your body's balance and what sets you off. More on that later.

The next 69 days are for everyone. I suggest looking at the most common meals you are currently eating and try to substitute with healthier options. Again, think less about the restrictions and more about the possibilities and newness of the food you're ingesting.

Things to avoid:

Wheat, barley, rye... gluten-ey things

Alcohol (a glass of red wine/stout beer is OK occasionally)

Caffeine

Farmed fish

Non-organic, non-grass fed, non-antibiotic free meat

Additives such as nitrates, sodium, MSG (monosodium glutamate)

High Fructose Corn Syrup

Margarine

Anything and everything fat-free or sugar-free

Anything in a can

Marinades or seasoning mixtures (i.e. Lowry's)

Clean eating. Whether you're getting back on track from a failed diet in the past or you're brand new, there is no substitute for food that is wholesome, nutritious and free from man-made substances. Items that are in the avoid sections contribute to a widespread phenomenon occurring mostly in developed nations called inflammation. In small amounts, your body processes and deals with it usually without issue. In large amounts, low-grade inflammation is directly linked to almost every chronic disease.

When you twist your ankle, it swells up and hurts a lot. You typically ice and have to stay off of it for several days to heal. This is a *severe* inflammatory response. Inflammation in the short-term is a good thing because it brings vital fluids and healing components to the area injured. Our bodies need a certain level of inflammation in order to heal from injuries and fight off acute disease and infection.

Inflammation in the long-term usually goes unnoticed by the person afflicted and if left untreated, can wreak havoc on the body in ways that are just now coming to light. Characteristics that encourage this kind of "under the radar" inflammation are high levels of stress, being overweight, poor diet, lack of exercise, toxin exposure and lack of restful sleep. Low-grade inflammation doesn't produce symptoms that are dramatic, and can linger under the surface for years.

There are cues that you should take note of that can indicate whether you are dealing with this. Take a close look at your life. Do you need coffee or caffeine to get you going in the morning? Do you feel tired no matter how much sleep you get? Do you have trouble with acne or eczema? Have you been told you have fibromyalgia, depression or inflammatory bowel disease? Are there times during the day you feel like there's a fog in your head? That's you... being inflamed. Turn the heat down. Allow your body to absorb nutrients efficiently and without difficulty. Chew your food for longer and take more time in between bites. Detox, baby. Detox.

If you have been told by nutritionists/doctors in the past to avoid certain foods or you should never do _____, I'm not telling you to ignore those recommendations. I will ask that you test and confirm their recommendations (unless you have life-threatening allergies). My father, for *years*, thought that he couldn't eat salads because his gastroenterologist said lettuce would inflame his ulcerative colitis. Every time my dad ate a salad, his UC would go nuts. 20 years later, he decided to try balsamic vinaigrette dressing versus his typical ranch. Hasn't had a problem since. Turns out he's lactose intolerant. The person with diverticulitis who can't eat seeds or high cholesterol who won't consume fats, keep an open mind and try something different.

As you move forward through the next 90 days, it will be very tempting to step on the scale every morning to check how much weight you have lost. It is the easiest guide to tell if you are doing well or not so well. I am going to challenge you to not step on the scale for these 90 days. Try not to get wrapped in numbers on a scale. Take my word for it and for 3 months ignore the scale. Use other markers for progress other than pounds lost or gained (or kilos for our metric friends). Do you feel like you have more energy? Do you have to shop for new clothes because your old clothes don't fit anymore? Do people ask you what you're doing different in your life because you look great! Or how about your skin? Is your skin clearer and healthier? These are more important indicators that will tell you that you are doing a great job and that the decisions you're making are having a huge impact on your health. Do you have to be 115 pounds to feel sexy or for people to notice? Of course not! I've said it before and I'll say it again, every step you take towards health is a win! Allow other indicators to steer you in the right direction. Your weight is just one indicator. Don't let one thing deter you from greatness in your life or make you feel like you haven't accomplished anything.

You're looking at 3 full months of establishing a foundation for your body to build on. A HUGE component to beginning something new is to plan ahead. Plan for snack time especially and have things on hand to munch that are nutritious and wholesome. For me, meal planning is make or break. If I do not have a plan for the day, it's straight to the junk. While take-out isn't horrible once in a while, if you're stuck between cooking something after a long day at work or calling for take-out and 30 minutes later getting dinner without dirty dishes... Which one wins? Fail to plan or plan to fail.

I get asked often about Cheat Days. Are there days that I can eat whatever I feel like and not feel bad about it? Of course, every day can be a cheat day if you want it to be and you shouldn't be made to feel bad about it. Your body will take on whatever habit you choose. Be cautious if you start to notice that your cheat days become more and more frequent until your cheat days outnumber the good decision days. Be flexible and realistic, but also be weary of the cheat day. Find a groove that works best for you because you will be doing this forever! Permanence is so important.

Keep in mind that if you start to re-introduce some foods and you notice a change in the way you feel or you have any kind of gastrointestinal upset, reconsider bringing that food back into your life. There have been many times when I haven't gone grocery shopping, so I'll eat whatever is left in the cupboard. Now understanding the needs of my own body, eating foods that don't agree with my chemistry will give me headaches, fatigue and serious, serious bloating. The first 2 you might not normally link to your diet. Keep a close eye on your journey through the next 3 months. There may be signs that something is wrong that get ignored because they are common in our culture. Headaches are common, but are they normal? Diarrhea and constipation may be common, but are they normal? Fatigue is an epidemic, but should that be the status quo?

I touched on this previously, but I can't stress enough how profoundly helpful it is to journal. The simple act of writing down how I was feeling on a certain day and what I ate correlates and brings to my attention connections that I might have missed without them being documented. If you notice that your heaviest cravings happen right when you get home from work, work on changing up that routine. Instead of going to the cupboard, head somewhere else instead. Journaling might grant insight into the inner workings of your body that you might be unaware of. Take three days and write down everything that goes into your mouth, good or bad. Have that be your baseline. Three months later, journal again for 3 days and see how you compare. Compare you to you! Not you to this book or you to anyone else. Notice the foods or items that have lingered and the amazing changes you have stuck with.

Write down symptoms you might be experiencing so you can better correlate those symptoms to foods you ate or something else in your day that might have contributed. It also makes the way you're feeling more manageable if you can pinpoint a cause. Sometimes an emotion can overtake our day and it's hard to focus on anything else, but if you compartmentalize and can understand why you might be feeling that way, it makes it smaller and more manageable.

While we are on the topic of symptoms, what should you do when you are experiencing symptoms like headaches or diarrhea? Let's return to our mission: to change the way we think and experience health. If you have a headache, it is easy to head over to the medicine cabinet and throw down some

Ibuprofen. For this, take that. *That's what needs to change*. In the beginning, you will be unsure of what's happening, therefore, you will not know which natural things you should do to alleviate the problem. It is your choice whether you want to continue taking things to change symptoms. I would advise you use caution when using over-the-counter medication to sort out your symptoms. Those symptoms are there for a reason: "God didn't make a shitty product." There is a process your body is going through. You will certainly feel better by taking OTC products, and that's okay to do as long as you're okay with it. Just for kicks, read every word on the box and insert of the medications you're using. Learn what you can before allowing those things to enter your body. Be picky about what enters your temple.

Another more science-y reason is that research often includes a test group and a control group. Let's say you have a headache. Your headache could be caused by dehydration, detoxification, a stroke or muscle tension or a vertebra that is out of alignment. If you take Tylenol, drink a liter of water and then go to get adjusted, what was it that helped? Your guess is as good as mine. Without a control group the results are useless. You have learned nothing other than your headache is no longer there. In the same situation, you have a headache and you look back on your journal and notice you only drank 12 fl oz of water or that it had been 4 weeks since your last adjustment. Now you not only have the solution to your current complaint, but can prevent future symptoms as well.

Some people would argue that it doesn't matter as long as the headache went away. That's the OLD way of thinking. No pain does not mean there isn't a problem. Lack of diagnosis does not mean lack of disease. Be your own best friend and try listening to your body instead of telling it what to do. It is talking to you all the time and taking the time to understand what's going on is a great way to reduce unnecessary prescriptions and OTC drug intake. Only a physician can advise you on whether you should stop taking your prescribed medication(s) and this book could never replace that advice, but you can start the conversation or ask questions. Help your doctor understand you. As mentioned earlier, these doctors have undergone years of training to do what they do, but there is no better expert in the study of your body than *you*. Don't ever forget that.

Chapter 7:

And Beyond...

As you complete these 90 days, you may feel a sense of dread or excitement. The dread stemming from a fear of what to do next. The excitement from either being done with the longest 90 days of your life or excitement that you made huge changes and saw incredible results!

Biggest Loser contestants often revert to their old habits after they return home because they weren't in the same controlled environment and lost their coaches. This last chapter you can read as many times as you like as you continue your journey. Consider this book, and me by proxy, your lifetime coach. The purpose of this book is to give you lifelong tools to address your lifestyle. While 90 days is a great start and the changes you have made will have long lasting effects, these changes are permanent and to continue on this path will require guidance now and again.

We discussed permanence in the second chapter. Accepting these habits as more than a fleeting moment of ambition and motivation. This is your new life. Get excited! This should be on the same level of awesome as driving a brand new car off the lot! You're driving in your new car every single day (hopefully not with the top down). Enjoy the new car smell, the pep in your step. Revel in all the moments, even the bad ones, that you experienced because they brought you to a different place.

If it has been months since your 90 days and you veered from your path, it's OK. The road gets a little bumpy and difficult to follow at times. If you remember that it is a path of your own creation and the turns and detours are only because of decisions you've made, you will find it easier and easier to get back on track. Maybe see those detours as scenic routes instead. Look back on those moments and know that you learned something about yourself that you can take with you. You are not weak; you are not incapable. Set standards that are worthy of your awesomeness. You are not a second class citizen. You are an inhabitant of your beautiful body with a mind steering you in any direction. You get to choose and you get to laugh at others who say you can't.

There might be things that come along that stand in your way. There may even be people in your life that disable you. Try to take those people with you on your journey. You might find the greatest support group ever are those who think they're just as weak and incapable. Be a leader amongst your friends and family and show them the path to true health that you have found. For those people that will not follow, who discourage, attack and undermine you (this might sting a little), but cut them out of your life. Surround yourself with people who want to make you better and lift you up. Do not give time to those who seek to destroy your work. The excision might not be permanent, but in this moment and at this time, you do not deserve to have people who suck the good energy out of you. You may invite them back as you see fit, but give them time to understand the commitment you've made to yourself and to your health.

Know that in every decision you made and every step towards health you took, I am infinitely and profoundly proud and inspired by you. I'm even more inspired by the times you felt the weakest and worst, but decided to change in spite of it! You cannot understand the greatness you hold inside until it is unleashed. Share that strength and insight with people you connect with and cross in your life. Who knows the number of lives *you* can change along with your own?

To shift your health, we must shift the paradigm.

You can be the change.

You can start a movement.

Recipes that don't make you hate cooking

Breakfast

Sweet Potato Omelet

1 Sweet Potato: shredded 2 Eggs

1/4 tsp cinnamon

Salt and Pepper

You can start a movement

Sautee everything together in coconut oil or grapeseed oil and serve.

Smoothies

Frozen fruit of any kind

1 banana

Ice

Fresh pressed juice or similar additive-free juice

Almonds

Put all ingredients in a blender and serve. After the first 2 weeks, you can add greek yogurt to the mix.

Sweet Fruit

A handful of assorted berries

1 tsp Cinnamon

1 Tbl Honey

A handful of almonds/pecans/walnuts

Put fruit and nuts in a bowl, sprinkle cinnamon, drizzle honey and eat it up.)

Coconut Porridge

2 Tbl almond butter

¼ C shredded coconut (unsweetened)

5 Tbl warm water

¼ tsp vanilla extract

½ tsp cinnamon

2 tsp honey

Pumpkin Porridge

1 Tbl tahini

½ can pumpkin puree

¼ C warm water

¼ tsp vanilla extract

½ tsp cinnamon

1 Tbl shredded coconut (unsweetened)

1 Tbl raisins/dried fruit

1 tsp honey

Snacks

Garlic Hummus

1 can Garbanzo beans (drained with about 1/2 c juice saved)

2 Tbl Tahini

2 Tbl Olive Oil

3 cloves garlic

1 tsp salt

1 tsp cumin

(red pepper flakes if you're into that)

Put it all in a blender and mix it up. Serve with veggies, tortilla chips, etc...

Nut Butter and Celery

Take a half empty jar of any kind of nut butter and stick stalks of cut-up celery in the jar. You can also add raisins. Ants on a log to go!

Energy Balls

1 C cooked and cooled steel-cut oats

½ C nut butter of your choice

½ C honey

1 tsp vanilla

½ C Flax seed, ground

½ C 70% or higher dark chocolate chips/chunks

Stuffed Mushrooms

12 Portobello mushroom caps

1 Tbl bacon fat/cooking fat

¼ C bell pepper, minced

¼ C red onion, minced

1 lb ground meat of your choice

2 C spinach, chopped fine

2 garlic cloves, minced

Preheat oven to 450° F. Bake mushrooms, caps down, for 10 minutes or until they start to weep.

In a large skillet, melt fat and sauté onion and peppers until onions are translucent. Add meat and cook through (about 5 minutes). Add spinach and garlic and stir together. Spoon the meat mixture into the mushroom caps and serve!

Tortilla Chips and Salsa

Organic salsa with all real ingredients that you can read and understand. Tortilla chips should be made from corn, oil and salt.

Lunch/Dinner

Spaghetti Squash Spaghetti

1 medium spaghetti squash: cut in half and de-seeded 5-6 medium tomatoes

1 Tbl Oregano

1 Tbl Basil

1-2 Bay Leaves

2-3 cloves garlic: minced

1 medium yellow onion: diced

Salt and pepper to taste

1 Tbl raw cocoa (optional)

Pre-heat oven to 350.

Lazy version: Place all ingredients except squash in a blender and blend. Put sauce in a pot, bring to a boil and then let simmer until you're ready to eat.

Ambitious version: Roast tomatoes at 350 for 10 minutes with salt before adding them to the blender. Cook spaghetti squash halves face down on a cookie sheet for 15-20 minutes and then scrape the insides with a fork (should resemble pasta). Serve sauce over squash.

In the 3rd week and beyond, you can add your favorite cooked meat choice to the simmering.

Pizza

4 cups cauliflower rice (blend up cauliflower until it looks like rice, steam for 10 minutes)

1 egg beaten

Some oregano

½ C to 1 C coconut flour

Tomato sauce

Veggies

Italian seasoning

(Meat if you're past the first 7 days)

Pre-heat oven to 350 degrees. Dump your cauliflower rice onto a dishtowel or absorbent rag, bundle it up like a hobo pack and squeeze the water out. You might need to do this one or two times with new towels to get the driest result. Mix together cauliflower, egg, oregano and flour until it looks like dough. Spread it to your thickness preference in a 9X9 or 9X12 and bake until golden brown. Add desired amount of tomato sauce, Italian seasoning, veggies and meat. Put back in the oven for 10-15 minutes. You can add hard cheese like sharp cheddar to the top for a more traditional-looking pizza.

Mac N' Cheese

1.5 heads of cauliflower chopped with leaves and head removed.

4 tbl Butter

½ tsp salt

¼ C Water

1 small yellow/summer squash cubed

1 small carrot diced

½ sweet onion diced

1 clove garlic

¾ tsp ground mustard

1 can coconut milk

1 egg

Pepper to taste

Cook cauliflower in 2 Tbl butter, ½ tsp salt and water in sauté pan for 5-6 minutes with a cover on. Remove from heat when florets are tender. Heat 2 tbl butter in a saucepan over medium heat. Add squash, carrot, onion, garlic clove, mustard and salt to pan and sauté until onions are translucent. Add the can of coconut milk and simmer for 10 minutes. Pour it all into a blender until well blended. Quickly add egg yolk and blend it up. Serve over cauliflower.

Fajitas

1 tbl coconut or avocado oil

3 peppers of assorted colors: sliced

1 medium onion: sliced or diced

1 medium summer squash: peeled and sliced or cubed

2 tsp cumin

1 tsp chili powder

Salt to taste

Fresh spring greens

Organic or homemade salsa

Red pepper flakes (if you're into that)

Gluten-free or corn tortillas

Sautee everything except greens and salsa in a pan until soft. Serve on tortillas with spring greens. You can substitute greek yogurt for sour cream and/or your choice of meat in week 3. You can also nix the tortilla and serve everything on a bed of greens.

Marinated Chicken Roll-up

2 Tbl lemon juice

2 Tbl minced garlic

2 tsp curry powder

1 tsp ground cumin

2 Tbl coconut/olive oil

1 lb chicken breast thinly sliced

Romaine lettuce leaves

Sauce

¾ C plain, whole fat Greek yogurt

¼ C tahini sauce/paste

1 Tbl minced garlic

2 tsp lemon zest + 1 Tbl lemon juice

Salt to taste

Get a large bowl and put first 5 ingredients in there. Add chicken to toss. Let sit 20-30 minutes (or overnight in the fridge) to marinate.

In a different bowl, whisk together all ingredients for the sauce.

Turn on the grill to medium-high and brush with some oil. Cook the chicken until it's cooked through. Serve with sauce on washed romaine leaves as roll-ups.

Yuuuuummy!

Here are where my numbers in the beginning chapters come from.

http://www.cms.gov/Research-Statistics-Data-and-Systems/Statistics-Trends-and-Reports/

NationalHealthExpendData/downloads/highlights.pdf http://kff.org/other/state-indicator/retail-rx-drugs-by-age/

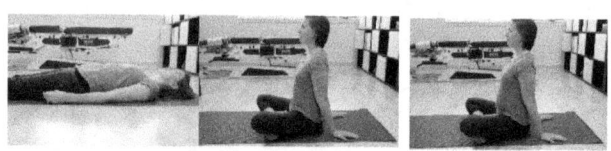

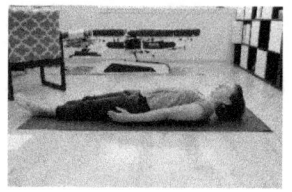

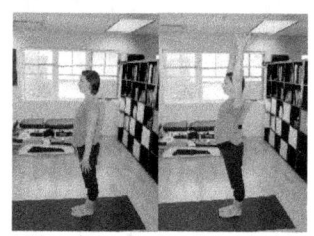

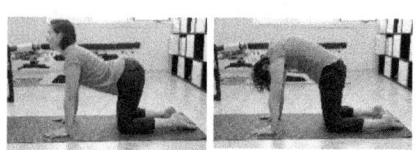

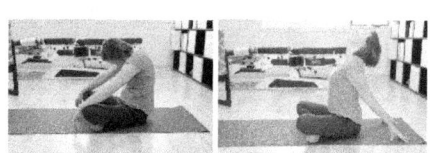

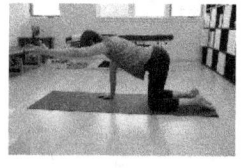

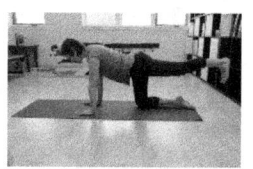

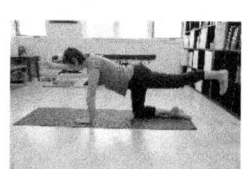

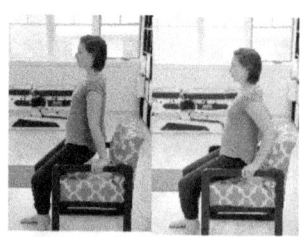

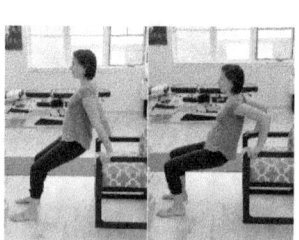

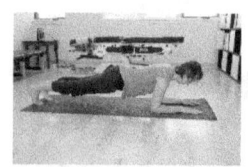

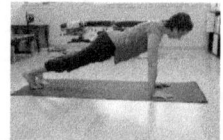

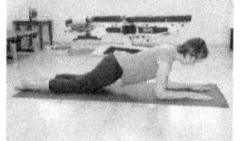

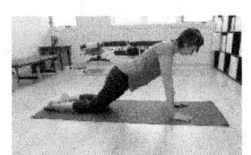 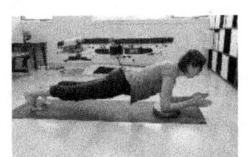 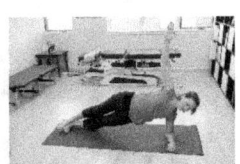

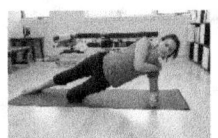 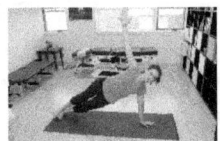

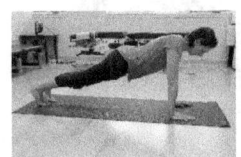 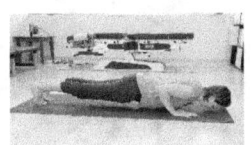 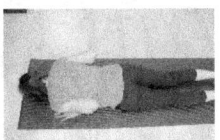

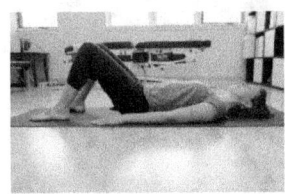 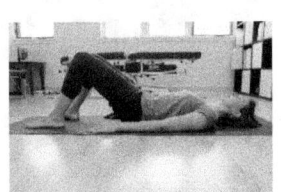

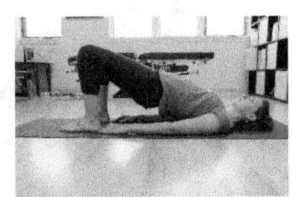 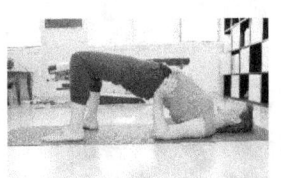

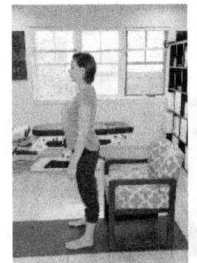 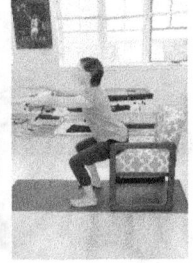 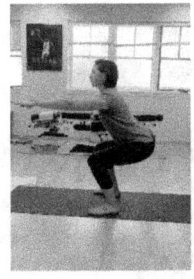

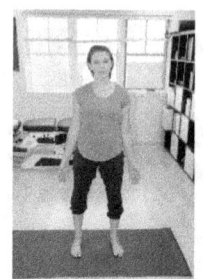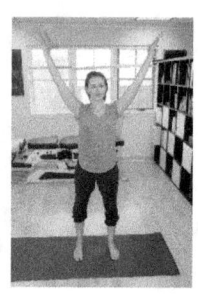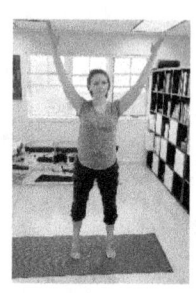

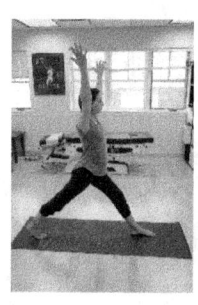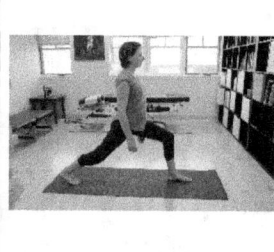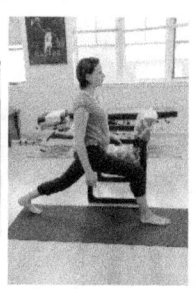

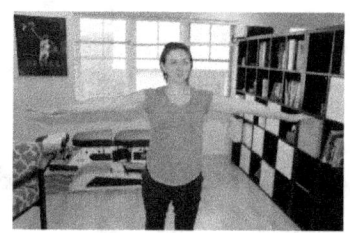

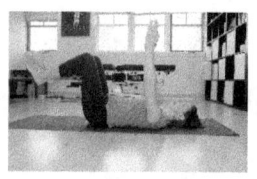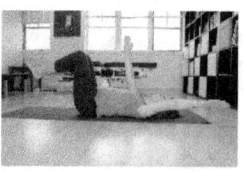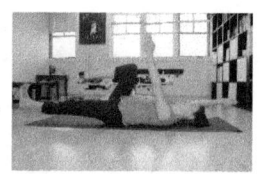

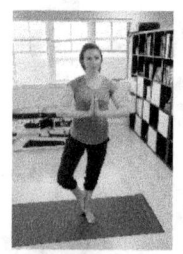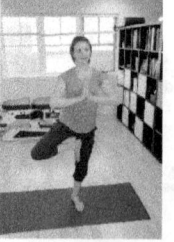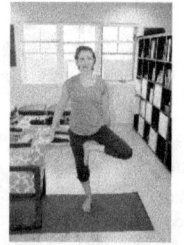

About the Author

I'm a chiropractor by day and mom, wife, chef, athlete and author by night (and the very, very early parts of the morning). After several years in practice, I realized there was more to health than a healthy spine. A healthy spine and functioning nervous system is a HUGE part of health, but my patients were coming in with all kinds of issues that their healthy spines couldn't support or heal.

Advocating for other people's health became my passion, my purpose and continues to be my reason for getting up in the morning.

While I'm not in the practice I share with my husband, I really enjoy yoga and being outdoors. It's my sanity. I've also found a CrossFit family here in Lake Forest that provides me with an incredible sense of community and support while I get my butt kicked in the workouts.

My 2 kids, Olivia (3 months) and Max (2.5 years) give me perspective. I value and appreciate them most for that. I didn't realize what it felt like to be selfish and selfless at the same time. They taught me how to achieve balance through learning and experimentation. It's for my family that I push myself. It's to show my kids, other young women, other professionals that ambition isn't selfish, happiness in work and home can be achieved and that dreaming big is never wasted.

My husband, Brandon, keeps me grounded. He's not only my anchor when my priorities shift, but he's also the goofy, thoughtful and supportive man I couldn't have even dreamt up.

And my parents and my sister: irreplaceable in my heart.